Unleash Your Inner Super Hero!

By Lauren Denos

ISBN-10:1482567776
ISBN-13:9781482567779

Cover Art by Natalie May

Dedications

This book is for those who are striving to become extraordinary. For those who seek to escape the mundane. The habits you form make you who you are. So create good ones!

Find your inner superhero, Strive for excellence and *LIVE FULL OUT!*

Special Thanks

Thank you to my awesome, hot, sweet man who puts up with me constantly thinking about work or some off the wall adventure. You are my sounding board and keep me sane when I need it. You help me to rest when I need it but can't see it. You keep my motorcycle in running condition, supply me with all the snuggles I could ever want, and accept my wild, free nature. I love you!

Thank you to my Mom, Dad and Brother who have been through so much with me. They saw all my distracted moments in life and supported me in anything I wanted to do. They were always there for me when I needed them. They always knew when I was in trouble even if I did not tell them and they would go to any length to help me. You gave me life at least three times and I am the person I am today because you pulled me out of the fire.

Thank you to all my wonderful friends who stick by me and give me great counsel to help me help others more. You have been such a great source of love in my life. You make my life rich.

Thank you to my Dynamic Fitness System community. You are the best! You always make me strive to be more. I love the support you all give to each other and me. You are all inspiring to me; you are all amazing!

Table of Contents

Steps To Making A Good Habit

Sticking To Your Guns

There's A Wall In My Way

Things To Remember

Introduction

*W*here are you today in your life? Are you where you want to be? Could you be more than you are now?

Most of us feel like we can be more or do more. Where you are now is because of the habits you have incorporated into your life and because of the ones you have never thought to develop.

Habits are the automatic things we do every day. And it is time for you to use them to your benefit!

I talk mostly in a health and fitness context in this book, but you can use these tools for every area in your life.

I wrote this book based on habits because I believe that we all have an inner superhero dying to get out. We have so much potential - we just need to tap into it. Good habits help the superhero in us emerge.

I want to help create a world where we all know we can accomplish anything and live the life we desire. I figure the best way to make this world I dream of a reality is to help mold it with what I have learned throughout my life so far.

I guess you could say **I am fighting mediocrity**.

We all have the potential to be superhero's but we have to want it and go for it no matter the set backs we face. Almost everyone in this world has faced adversity. The trick is to unleash your inner superhero and not let the adversity hold you back. Discover your inner superhero today and live the life you desire!

Kick ass, take names and LIVE FULL OUT!

Lauren Denos

We Are Creating Habits Every Day.

"We are what we repeatedly do. Excellence, then, is not an act, but a habit."

~ Will Durant on Aristotle

Before we jump into how to create habits, it is important to know what a habit is.

Habits: Automatic routines of behavior and thoughts that are repeated regularly, without conscious thought. These are learned behaviors and are not instinctive.

It is also important to note which habits are **healthy** or **unhealthy.**

Healthy habits include:

- Going to the gym everyday and working out

- Brushing your teeth morning and night

- Drinking water when you are thirsty

- Putting your seat belt on

Unhealthy habits include:

- Smoking

- Drinking soda

- Grabbing candy every time you go by the candy bowl

- Getting pizza every Monday

What habits would you like to create?

_____
_____
_____
_____
_____
_____
_____
_____

To create a habit, you must first:

MAKE A CONSCIOUS DECISION TO WANT TO CHANGE THIS PART OF YOUR LIFE.

Once you've made the decision to want to change, developing the habit is the easy part. Now lets move on to starting the process.

Part 1

The Steps to Making a Habit

Identify Your Goals

"People with goals succeed because they know where they're going."

~ Earl Nightingale

*B*efore you can do anything to create your new habit you need to know what your goal is.

Do you want to gain muscle mass, lose body fat, lower your blood pressure to decrease your risk of a heart attack, or leap tall buildings?

You can get a personal trainer to help you with a plan or research how to start on your own.

What you want to do will determine the goal you set. If you want to bulk up and have more muscle mass then you are going to want to make a habit of heavy weight training.

If your goal is to be a better runner you are going to want to make a habit of running, weight training and maybe plyometrics (Plyometrics are explosive movements that can help athletes improve their game).

If your goal is to eat better, you are probably going to want to make a habit of planning and prepping your meals daily.

There are so many tools and techniques for goal setting, Since we are focusing on creating better habits in this book we will keep the goal setting part simple and easy. Choose one goal and make sure when you are choosing your goal that you use these techniques.

1. Be specific! The more detailed the better.

Non-Specific Goal Setting: "I want to be in better shape."

Specific Goal Setting: "I want to lose 4 inches off my waist."

Specificity is so important - without it we don't really know what we want, we just have a blurry idea. Lets say you want to go to a concert, so that is what you ask for. Suddenly your friend surprises you with tickets to a Celine Deon concert, but you don't actually like that kind of music and wanted something like Tool or Zac Brown Band. Well, at that point you can not complain because your friend gave you what you asked for. Now, if you would have said, "I would like to go to a Tool or a Zac Brown Band concert", you would have been more likely to get what you wanted, or something closer to it. Be specific!

2. Make it measurable.

It is important to record our results so we can see the progress we've made. An example is: Measure your body with a tape measure or time your runs, you could also keep track of the distance you run.

Making your goal something you can measure will let you know that you are actually on target. If you are like me and wear spandex all the time, then you may have a hard time knowing if you are gaining or losing weight unless you measure yourself. That could be bad. You need to see the progress you are making so that you can know you are on the right track; besides, it helps motivate you to see the goal through to completion. So what ever it is, make sure you can measure it! It could be a check list for your healthy meals, to make sure you ate what you were supposed to each day; it could be a log of how many pushups you do. What ever your goals are, find a way to make them measurable; this will help a lot!

A note of caution- Throw your damn scale away! Do not use it as your source of measurement. Scales do not take into account the amount of muscle verses fat in your body. So you could be losing inches and becoming more compact and yet the scale could be going up. The scale can be a mind game and can tend to make people crazy! Just stop! Use a better method, such as body fat testing or cloth measuring tape - or just how your jeans are fitting. If you are dealing with a health professional they may use multiple measurement tools. If they are using a scale along with body fat testing and measurements to see what is going on in the body that is fine. But to use the scale as your only measurement of how you are doing with your health goals, you will drive yourself crazy. The scale alone it is not an accurate gauge.

3. Make it Attainable

It is crucial to be realistic when setting goals.

I speak from experience when I say that it is not the best feeling in the world when you have your heart set on a huge goal, and then not succeed at accomplishing it.

There is nothing wrong with stretching yourself, But you want to make it something that is attainable and more importantly something you BELIEVE you can achieve. When you say, "I am going to be a fitness model in two months", yet you are currently sitting at 50% body fat, that may be setting yourself up for a disappointment, and then it is easy to give up on all of your goal setting. Now, can you achieve being a fitness model? Of course you can! But be realistic on how long it will take and what it will take to get there. I like to create some goals that are so simple I know I will accomplish them with ease; it gives me some momentum. Then, I have the ones that are going to require more effort and work but are still doable. As you do more and more of the goal setting, you will stretch yourself further, but for now make sure it is something you can really accomplish.

If you have a big crazy goal, great, keep it! But break it down into some smaller, more easily attainable, goals. This way you are saying it is possible, but you are breaking it down into bite sizes so that you do not feel overwhelmed.

4. Put a time limit on your goal.

When do you want to accomplish it by? Remember to be specific and realistic.

Have you ever had a friend who talks about what they are going to do, but they never really set a date, and it just keeps getting pushed further and further into the future? They talk about how they are planning to go back to school, or someday they are going to be a famous stunt car driver , yet they never accomplish it and you hear about it for years. The reason is: if we do not have a deadline on something, we will keep pushing it in the future, and we do not see anything wrong with that.

Time flies by and you will not even realize how much time has passed, until one day you wake up and you realize all the dreams you had have not been accomplished yet.

Put a deadline on your goals. Put them up in your house so they are in front of your face so you can not push them away or hide from them.

List a goal or two that you are thinking you would like to create habits for.

_____

_____

_____

5. Make sure you are setting the goals YOU want to achieve.

Look at your goals for a moment. Answer the following:

What do you want?

_____
_____
_____
_____
_____

Why do you want it?

_____
_____
_____
_____
_____

What will this change in your life?

_____
_____
_____
_____
_____

Why have you not done anything towards this before?

_____
_____
_____
_____
_____

Where did this goal come from?

_____

_____

_____

_____

_____

Is this what you want, or what others have pushed on you?

_____

_____

_____

_____

_____

The answers to these questions are important. They tell you if the person you are working towards becoming is who you really want to be, or if you are working towards fitting a mold that you haven't chosen for yourself.

If you find that you are working towards fitting a mold, you are more likely to get off track. Keep it focused on what YOU really want.

Superheros are true to themselves and do not attempt to be anything else. They do what they know to be correct not what others tell them to do. That is a great lesson that we can learn from them.

After asking these questions about your goals which one have you decided are the right ones for you?

_____

Write Out Your Goals

"Goals that are not written down are just wishes." ~ Fitzhugh Doson

Write out your goals. This cements them into your head and makes them more real. It also clarifies them and gives you more of an idea of how to accomplish them. You can either look at this piece of paper every day or, my favorite, write it again everyday. Not only will this drill it deeper into you, but you will grow and expand upon it as you write it to make it more and more complete and detailed.

To start, write your big goal in a positive way, Such as: I am a marathon runner instead of I am not lazy anymore, or I am no longer a bad runner. Do you see how you want to make the goal positive? Something you are aiming for instead of something you are pushing away from? Also write your goal as if you are already achieving it. Then below it write how you are accomplishing it. Establish a date of achievement for this goal.

Look at what you are aiming to accomplish and create

your goals from that. For example if you are going to run 3 miles a day that in itself could be a habit you are going to create. It would be even better to say I am going to start running a minimum of 3 miles a day after work. This way you have your time laid out. Or maybe if you are going to be eating better then you would make a habit of prepping your meals each day for the following day when you are making dinner.

For example, let's say I want to complete a marathon. I could state my goal this way:

I am a marathon runner

Goal:

I will run a full marathon by August 23rd of this year

I am achieving this by:

- Running at least 3 miles a day for one month. 5 miles a day on month 2. and continue this pattern.

- Eating protein and veggies at each meal, and eat healthy carbohydrates.

My habit I am creating is:

- Running a minimum of 3 miles a day as soon as I get home from work.

- Prepping my healthy balanced meals each night when I make dinner.

If you create a goal like running a marathon, weight training will also be very helpful to build the muscles that will give you more stamina and power for your running.

Goal:

_____

_____

Date I will accomplish this : _____

I am achieving this by:

_____
_____
_____
_____
_____
_____
_____
_____
_____
_____

The Habit I will create to achieve this is

_____
_____
_____
_____
_____
_____
_____
_____

Know the Benefits and Consequences

"It seems, in fact, as though the second half of a man's life is made up of nothing but the habits he has accumulated during the first half." ~ Fyodor Mikhailovich Dostoevsky

Knowing all the reasons of why you are creating a habit is a good thing to help keep you on track.

Write yourself a list. You can rewrite this list daily with your goals if you like.

List at least 5 things that will happen if you succeed at this goal, and 5 things that may happen if you fail at this goal. These reasons need to be very meaningful to you. The more you dig for deep meaning reasons, the easier it will be to stay on track and motivated.

Anytime you feel like bailing out of your good new habit, look at the list of reasons why you wanted to create this habit.

The benefits of exercise are an endless list of positives. Perhaps you simply want to lose weight and look better, or maybe there are health issues that will be resolved by following this healthier lifestyle. Example: Let's say your goal is to eat a clean diet full of lean meat, veggies and fruits, and limit sugar, breads, and dairy. (some people are fine with breads and sugars and some are not, this is an example for those who have issues with breads and sugars)

The Good Stuff

1. I will automatically start leaning down

2. I will have more energy

3. I will reverse my insulin resistance

4. I will be focused with a clear head

5. I will sleep better at night

The Bad Stuff

1. I will have headaches and stomach pains

2. I will have to buy bigger clothing (no longer fitting into my super spandex suit)

3. People may judge me

4. I will feel like a failure

5. I will be sluggish and unable to do what I want

Your turn

The Good Stuff

_____
_____
_____
_____
_____
_____
_____
_____
_____
_____

The Bad Stuff

_____
_____
_____
_____
_____
_____
_____
_____
_____
_____

Start the Journey!

"A journey of a thousand miles must begin with a single step." ~ Lao Tzu

*I*t takes about 30 days for something to become a habit.

Commit to the 30 days. For some people it takes a longer or shorter amount of time, but 30 days is a general rule of thumb.

Decide what positive habit you want to start. It could be drinking more water, taking a yoga class, walking or jogging everyday, eating healthier, starting to lift weights or breaking the sound barrier. You should have an idea of what habit you would like to create from the exercises you have done in previous chapters.

What is this new habit?

_____

Be prepared. You want to give yourself all the help you can to remember and be motivated to do this. Maybe you set your gym clothes on the edge of your bed or next to the coffee pot, Or maybe you have a friend that you can team up with. You can call each other every morning to remind each other to get to the gym.

What can you do to prepare better to make this new habit easier to stick with?

_____
_____
_____
_____
_____
_____

Once you decide which habit you are going to build, another option is to start a 30 day group. You can do this a few different ways:

- One way is to get a group of people together who want to change a habit, <u>any</u> habit in their lives, and make it a 30 day support group to help each other accomplish their goals.

- Another way is to find people who want to accomplish a similar goal, such as running every morning. With this type of group, you have people who can meet up and run with you. This can be one of the best groups to have.

Or, if you are not particular about the type of exercise you want to do, just create a workout group; each person can take a turn at creating a routine for everyone.

You could create a group that meets in person once a week, or you could do an online group. When you have a group like this, you can talk about what is working and what is not working, and help each other in the new habit process. Doing this will help each other be accountable and to cheer each other on!

For thirty days you: **commit to the challenge**, have a check in, either by email, online or in person. This provides the accountability and you can report your successes. This is a really great feeling of reward when you get to report that you kept your commitment. You could check in as little as once a week, I would recommend you check-in every day, if you can, you are far more likely to stick with it when you have the daily accountability.

There is also the value of reporting your struggles. Your teammates will help encourage you to stick to your new habit and support you through your struggles.

Even Superheroes work in teams. If it helps them, it can help you too.

When you see everyone else doing great in their goals, it's really inspiring!

If they can do it, so can I! We're all in this together.

A couple of guidelines:

1. Choose an easy goal. Don't decide to do something really complex, at least for now. Later, when you've done this and know what it takes, you can choose something intense. But for now, do something you know you can do every day. The success in this will help you develop a rhythm and propel you forward.

2. Choose something measurable. You should be able to say, definitely, whether you were successful or not each day. If you choose exercise, set a number of minutes, or something similar (20 minutes of exercise daily). Whatever your habit, have a tangible measurement.

3. Be consistent. You want to work on your new habit at the same time every day, if possible. If you're going to exercise, you could do it at 7 am. (or 6 pm.) every day, for example. This makes it more likely to become a habit. It is nice if you have the flexibility in your schedule to do this at the same time every day. But if not, still work on your new habit during whatever time of the day you have.

List 10 people that you can call to create a group for creating habits

_____

_____

_____

_____

_____

_____

_____

_____

_____

_____

Call your support team and get it going. You can develop healthy habits on your own, but a group is a great way to stay motivated. You do not have to have 10 people to start a group, you can do this with just one other person. The point is if you call 10 people you should get at least a few people who are interested. If you get all 10 that is great too. The more minds working together the better!

Committing to Yourself

"There is a difference between interest and commitment. When you're interested in doing something, you do it when circumstances permit. When you're committed to something, you accept no excuses, only results." ~ Anonymous

Take little steps.

Start with 10-30 minutes of weight training or cardio and work up from there. Don't do so much that you get burned out really fast.

Remember, we are aiming for the long term.

If you start out with an hour of heavy weights or intense cardio you may find it too stressing and decide that it is just not worth it. Getting to the gym will be a great accomplishment, and keep you going.

You may have heard the saying "It's the little things in life that count". Well that certainly is the truth with health and fitness. All the little things will add up and make a big contribution to your well-being.

Simple things like parking further away from the grocery store or walking to the deli from work can add up to make a difference. Find the little things in your day that will add up to make a healthy impact.

Consistency with this makes all the difference. If a superhero was sometimes around to save the day and other times not there when you need them, would you keep trusting them? In order for you to believe in yourself and what you are doing you need to stay consistent too.

Remember you are your own superhero, be there for yourself and be consistent. This does not mean that you will be perfect with no slip ups, but it will help that you will get back up when you fall and that you keep going. Commit to yourself. You will make this change!

What small thing can you commit to doing on a regular basis?

_____
_____
_____
_____
_____

Start Slow

"A habit cannot be tossed out the window; it must be coaxed down the stairs a step at a time." ~ Mark Twain

*I*t is more important that you are starting this habit, than how fast you are getting going. For so many of us just the act of getting out for a 10 minute walk or getting to the gym, Small steps lead to big leaps.

Start slow and grow from there. If you have decided to go workout at a gym, to workout at home or outdoors, either way you need to take it slow and gradual, but be consistent.

Get your routine planned and start at a comfortable pace.

Even superheroes have a training period when they are first getting started on their path. They have to train and get good at their healthy habits and their job of saving lives.

We are living in a quick fix society. We want everything at the touch of a button and we want it instantly! Many people do this with their health, but most have only temporary success and then they find themselves shortly after in a worse place than when they started. The reason for this is that it did not become a lifestyle. When we slowly add things to our lives and get use to it before we move on then we build a habit, then we can build upon that. So when you are working on your health ask yourself if you would rather take it slow and make it stick or do you want the temporary fix and end up yo-yoing to nowhere?

If you have been wanting to get in shape then look at what you want to accomplish and then break it down into the small things you can do and then take it slow and learn to enjoy the journey you are on. One very important thing I have learned from clients and with myself is that there is no magical point that we suddenly become happy. How many times have you heard someone else or yourself say "when I loose 20 pounds then I will be happy"? But it does not really work that way. Because once we get there we realize what else we have not accomplished yet. That elusive happiness just keeps getting pushed further and further into the future. instead realize that this is a journey, you will continue to get better and better and this process will continue. So be happy with what you have now and breath. Take slow steps, be patient and they will become life long habits.

If you eat the typical American diet of fast food, tons of sugar and soda then a good example of a huge step would be:

- I want to have a perfectly clean diet. Only lean meats and veggies for every meal!

You make this smaller steps like this:

- Reduce soda intake to 1 a day

- cook dinner at home

- choose healthier solutions at the fast food place

Have you been thinking in huge steps? What is it?

_____

Now how can you break this down into small steps?

_____
_____
_____
_____
_____
_____
_____

Create Reminders

"Winning is a habit. Unfortunately, so is losing." ~ Vince Lombardi

I use index cards or post it notes often and post them up all over where I will see them. I put things like: go do your bike ride at 12:00pm or Prep your food at 8:00pm.

A screen that pops up on your computer as soon as you open it can be a great reminder. Also having a buddy as mentioned in other chapters works well too, it creates an accountability that is outside of yourself, making it harder to get out of.

Pack your gear bag the night before. Workout clothes, shoes, water, etc. and set it by the door or in your car. This way, if you are rushed in the morning, this task is already completed and you will still get to your scheduled workout.

Your reminders can range anywhere from hanging up your skinny jeans so you can see them daily, to taping a picture of a bikini model on your refrigerator, You can make a fake magazine cover with your face on a bikini models body, to writing yourself post it notes, to setting out your work out clothes, you name it. What ever works for you.

Make sure which ever method you choose to use is a positive one. If you are using the bikini model picture then make sure you are seeing that as a positive reminder to be the best you can be and not as a way to feel bad about yourself.

Reminders are very important since we are so busy being superheroes in other areas of our lives that when we are creating a new habit things can be forgotten.

Do not leave this to chance!

Create your reminders and prep things ahead of time so nothing stands in your way.

What reminders do you think would be great motivation for you? List at least 5 things

_____

_____

_____

_____

_____

_____

_____

_____

_____

_____

Being Consistent

Make your new habit as consistent as possible. If you make it at the same time of day at the same place it creates more of an automatic response.

Now I know that many people, myself included get bored going to the same place all the time. If you are one of those people then you may want to create a schedule that has different activities.

Keep those consistent too (for now).

If you are going to jog the park Monday make it every Monday at the same time. Maybe you go kayaking on Tuesday. Just make sure it is the same place and time every Tuesday.

The point here is that you have what you're going to do already planned out. This way, you do not need to think each day, "What do I want to do today?" That kind of thinking does not create a habit. In fact thinking like this many times does not even get you to workout that day.

The great thing is once you are consistent and your habit is formed you can switch things up a bit. So let's say you have your schedule, run on Mondays and Thursday, Gym Tuesday and Fridays, and Wednesday is swimming at the lake. You could easily change up locations and decided to go swim twice one week and run once etc. Having the schedule will keep you from thinking too hard about it and possibly missing your workout all together, but there is nothing wrong with changing things up as long as you stay consistent with the workouts. Variety keeps your workouts fun and interesting, this keeps you going, just also make it consistent.

Now, consistency isn't really the sexiest or most exciting thing in the world, but with time it will give you real results in your life.

Sticking with the program and doing something consistently, and not just when you feel inspired, is very powerful. This is what a habit is.

Create your list of what you will be doing and on what days, and preferably what time.

*Monday*_____

_____

_____

_____

*Tuesday*_____

_____

_____

_____

*Wednesday*_____

_____

_____

_____

*Thursday*_____

_____

_____

_____

*Friday*_____

_____

_____

_____

*Saturday*_____

_____

_____

_____

*Sunday*_____

_____

_____

_____

Incorporate Friends

"Individuals play the game, but teams beat the odds." ~ SEAL Team saying

Yes, I said this already. It warrants saying it again. A commitment buddy can make such a big difference. No matter what you do.

I have workout buddies, accountability buddies and business buddies It helps me to stay committed and gives me an extra "oomph" when I am tired and would just rather stay home and veg.

I have a mastermind group that I meet with twice a month where we declare our goals and get specific about it. If we do not accomplish them there are consequences. This group helps so much with anything I want to accomplish in business, health or personal. This can be a great tool, And you can create your own.

To create a mastermind group, I like to first off find people who have qualities that I would like to have. So if you want to be better in business find people who are great in business, if you want to get in better shape find people who have the bodies you like, If you want to learn new Super abilities find people who fly, go invisible and have super strength and the like. Invite about 4-8 people to this group. You can meet in person or do conference calls. I personally like meeting in person. In this group you have the minds of all of the other people to help you solve issues as they come up.

You set your goals and intentions for the week. And if you do not accomplish them you have some sort of consequence, for instance maybe $10 in the community funds. Or if $10 means nothing to you make it $100. Or you could commit to cleaning one of the other group members houses if you do not accomplish your goals. Whatever you make it, just make sure it is something that is enough of a consequence that it pushes you.

You can read more on how to create a mastermind group by reading Think and Grow Rich by Napoleon Hill, he has a whole chapter in his book about mastermind groups. And then focus it more on health, if that is what you are aiming for, which I assume since you are reading this.

What people could you call to create accountability or groups with? I am sure you can use the people from the list you made in previous sections.

_____
_____
_____
_____
_____
_____
_____
_____

Replace What You are Getting Rid of

"A nail is driven out by another nail. Habit is overcome by habit." ~ Desiderius Erasmus

Replacing what you are getting rid of works a couple of ways. It can be that you need to rearrange things so that you are not unbalancing your life too much such as if you need to wake up earlier to get to the gym, then maybe you want to go to bed a little earlier.

If you are working out in the evening and it is cutting into your time with a loved one then maybe you can make them your workout partner, or spend a little more quality time together on the weekend.

In this way we make sure that we are not neglecting things that are important. Whenever we start something new we are taking that time from somewhere. So it important to see how we can balance it out.

The second way we replace what we are getting rid of is when we are wanting to get rid of an old bad habit. The best way to get rid of a bad habit is to replace it with a good one.

Some examples are:

- If you feel some emotional eating "kicking in" recognize it and replace it. Find other "treats" you can replace that with or supplement an activity like going for a walk.

- Replacing your caramel, heavy whip coffee with a regular cappuccino or a tea

- Instead of a normal date night of pizza and a movie replace it with a healthier meal and bowling

If you get rid of something in your life and do not replace it with something else there is more of a chance of going back to the bad habit or whatever it is that you wanted to get rid of. This is why many smokers take up chewing on straws or eating hard candy. They have to have something to replace that habit with and they may repeat the process a few times so that they can first get off the cigarettes and then get off the hard candy and then get off of chewing straws. They can keep progressing this until they have a healthy habit that they can live with.

What bad habit would you like to replace? This can be a habit of eating ice cream in the middle of the night or smoking. It can be small or big but they are all important.

So how about it? What bad habit do you want to get rid of and what can you replace it with?

Do Not Have an Expectation on the Outcome

"Do not have an expectation on the outcome. Be firm on the principle but flexible on the method." ~ Zig Ziglar

Just give it a month and see what happens. You are not a failure if it does not work, you just did it a certain way to test it out. If that does not workout do it another way until you find the way that works for you. We can have a positive attitude and really see ourselves accomplishing our goal but do not hold onto exactly how it will happen. We never know exactly how things are going to play out. That's the fun part about living life! It may take once or may take 5 or more times until we find the magical combination that works for us. This way you can see it as a game and have fun with it verses stressed out about it.

Remember always enjoy the journey you are on no matter where that journey may lead you. Life is about the experiences you have along the way just as much as the actual destination of your trip.

Focus on today. One day at a time, making healthy food choices and getting today's workout done. Whether your goal is to run a lap around the planet or walk one mile, just get today's objective done.

What successes towards you goals did you have today?

_____
_____
_____
_____
_____
_____
_____
_____

You can journal this everyday if you like to see the successes you have had to keep you on your 30 day stretch.

You can also journal what the challenges you had today and how you can overcome them better next time.

Part 2

Sticking to Your Guns!

Take It Very Personally

"Your time is limited, so don't waste it living someone else's life. Don't be trapped by dogma- which is living with the results of other people's thinking. Don't let the noise of others opinions drown out your own inner voice. And most important, have the courage to follow your heart and intuition. They somehow already know what you truly want to become. Everything else is secondary."

~ Steve Jobs

$\mathcal{M}$ake sure that you are doing this for yourself. Do what is right for you. Be sure your workouts and your nutrition plan are personal to you. No one else is going to know exactly what you like or exactly what is right for you. If you are working with a personal trainer or coach then they will have some ideas on how to get you to where you want to go, but still the choice is ultimately yours and only you know what is going on in you.

For example, if you join the gym, do your personal workout with your routine. You don't have to keep up with everyone else in the gym, you can go at your own pace and do what is effective for you. If you do a group class, be sure to pick one that is appropriate for your level. Don't join Super Insane Turbo Kick if you have never taken a kick boxing class. Find what is appropriate for your fitness level.

Also find what you like. If you hate being in the gym then don't go to the gym! Go hiking, kayaking, running, play tennis, etc. Just make sure you are doing what you want to do. You may even want to test out a lot of exercises and sports before you find the one or few that is right for you. Do what you like and you will keep doing it.

What type of activities do you like to do or have wanted to test out?

_____
_____
_____
_____
_____

Wavering Path

"Success is a journey, not a destination."
~ Anonymous

Pretty much nothing in life is as simple as getting from point A to point B.

We are on a path that wavers and sometimes goes in a completely different direction. We can course correct and get back on target at any time. And we will have to do that to stay on target.

I myself have had so many distractions come up and different paths open up and then taken the long way around to get to a certain destination in my life.

If we have an idea of where we want to go and remain flexible on how we get there, we will get there. There are many paths to the top of the mountain.

If you have taken a break from exercise either because of life, or illness or surgery, here are some ideas to help you get back into it.

1. Take a photo of yourself from all different angles in you bathing suit or sports bra and underwear. When you fall off the wagon, look at the pictures and it should motivate you to keep going. (Only if this is a positive motivation for you).

2. Take it easy at first. Don't go right back to your heavier weights, or push yourself to the limit in cardio. Once you're back into your routine, then you can push harder again.

3. Do exercises you really enjoy. Get creative. Plan to meet somebody at the gym. Or go swimming. Make it fun again!

4. Plan after work walk or run dates, instead of after work drinks, It's healthier and can be fun.

5. Look at your goal list and Pro's and Con's list. Remember why you are doing this. It is a journey, not perfection.

6. Take a picture of yourself either in your favorite superhero outfit or put your face on your favorite superhero body! That way you will remember the superhero waiting to come out!

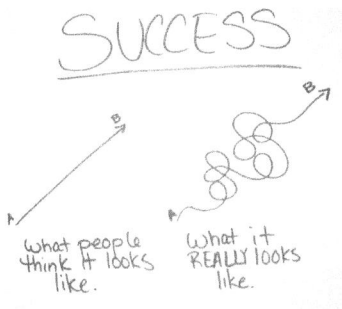

Part 3

There's a Wall in my Way!

Road Blocks

"A successful man is one who can lay a firm foundation with the bricks others have thrown at him."~ David Brinkley

Road blocks can be anything. They can be physical, emotional, and they can even, once in a while, be something out of our control.

There are unlimited types of road blocks, some examples of road blocks could be:

- Getting depressed because you are not seeing results fast enough.

- You injured your body.

- Or that you have NO healthy food in the house.

You can overcome or go around all of these.

First of all a block or obstacle only happens when you have momentum. We can not come up to blocks if we are stagnant. Should you come across obstacles, and you start to think that you are not getting anywhere, remember this:

If you were not moving forward you would not have come across the obstacle at all.

Obstacles are a part of life. It can be difficult to determine what to do to move forward. How do you know if you go over or around the wall? Honestly...you already know the answer within yourself. All answers lie inside us. You just have to know how to access the answers.

The first thing to do is STOP doing the activity that gets you hitting the wall. You will only frustrate yourself more in doing this and the more frustrated you get, the more likely you are to quit.

Now you need to go back through the steps you were taking and figure out at what point your progress stopped. Look at what the obstacle is. Is it something simple or is it something much more complicated?

Typically these are just obstacles placed in our path to teach us something, sometimes nothing more than "patience". You will be annoyed by the delay but you will be able to carry on.

Obstacles can be a sign that you are moving forward and they can make us stronger. I would recommend starting to embrace these challenges because many times when you stop having so many it means you have slowed down your learning in life.

Get out of your mind and search your inner wisdom. One of the biggest issues we have when overcoming obstacles is ourselves.

You might also need to step away from the situation and take a walk or get some fresh air. Many of us get into sensory overload, and getting some mellow introspective time can yield the answers you need without the stress. Besides it is important to get outside every once in a while to enjoy a stroll in the sun or relax. How are you going to recharge your powers otherwise?

"Quitters never win and Winners NEVER quit!"

List road blocks that could come up. Think of as many as you can. And they can be as wild and out there as you want.

Road blocks

_____
_____
_____
_____
_____
_____
_____
_____
_____
_____
_____
_____
_____

Look For Solutions

"There's no use talking about the problem unless you talk about the solution."

~ Betty Williams

Once you have identified what the block is, stop stressing about it and start looking for the solutions to the issue. Let's say you have sprained your ankle and your habit is to be running everyday.

Okay we already know what the problem is but harping on it will only make you feel worse and is counter productive. Now the next step is figuring out the solution to this issue. How can you get around the sprained ankle and stick with your new habit?

- If you are in a wheel chair from the sprain you can wheel yourself around instead of running

- You can work the supporting muscles in the gym during that time instead

- You can concentrate on your upper body

I know that these are not exactly running, but they will support your habit and once your ankle is better your body will be even further along.

Yes, this is an extreme example but the point is that you need to be a solution finder instead of a problem dweller. This is a big difference between Superheroes who succeed and those who fail, and superheroes never fail. They keep getting up until they succeed.

For each block you listed in the previous chapter find at least one solution. The more solutions you find for each block the better you will be able to handle any situation that comes your way.

Now take those road blocks from above and here we will find solutions to them.

Solutions

_____
_____
_____
_____
_____
_____
_____
_____
_____
_____
_____
_____
_____

Climbing the Wall

"Problems are only opportunities with thorns on them."~ Hugh Miller

One of the ways to deal with certain blocks we have towards fitness and health is to just do it! By this I mean get started with what you can.

If you have a block coming up with your cardio and you always seem to have a reason you can not do it then if going for a walk gets you started, then you have worked through one block. Keep up the walking and then add in some light jogging and then eventually some sprints. Tada! You have worked through that block.

As you do this you may have things that come up for you mentally, pay attention to them. These thoughts and beliefs that come up may help you figure out why this is an issue for you.

Little by little you will be getting through the barriers.

Let's say that your new habit is getting to the gym everyday. But you are having some sort of block coming up that is keeping you from getting to the gym. Maybe it is that you are too busy or that you just don't have the energy. Instead of worrying about getting the gym for an hour or even a half hour go for 10 minutes. If after that 10 minutes you feel like doing more then great! But even if it is only 10 minutes you have still officially gotten through one block!

What is a block that has been keeping you from creating your new habit? And what small step can you take to get the ball rolling?

_____

_____

_____

_____

_____

_____

_____

_____

_____

_____

_____

Move Through Your Excuses!

"Excuses are the nails used to build a house of failure."~ Don Wilder

An excuse is a defense or justification for something that would otherwise not be acceptable.

An excuse is something we tell ourselves or others to excuse ourselves from doing or accomplishing what needs to be done.

I think it's safe to say all of us have used excuses. Have you ever said "I don't have time to workout because I am too busy"? Or how about "I don't have money to join a gym or hire a trainer so I can't workout"?

These are just excuses.

Do you need tons of time to get in a workout? No! You could do a 10 minute routine. Do you have to have a gym membership or a trainer to workout? No! There are TONS of free resources out there. And there is always your house and the good old outdoors to use for your workouts!

Could you see a Superhero saying "yeah, I would love to come and save your life and battle the bad guy, but I'm kinda sore and really beat. Can we do this another day?"NO! Because they know excuses are just ways to avoid what we know needs to get done. It is easier to just do it! Then it is done and you are stronger for it.

First, acknowledge the excuses, and then see if you can figure out what the reason is behind the excuse and then find a way to move through it.

One of mine was not feeling well too often. I would be either getting sick or just not feeling good and then I would let myself sleep in instead of going to the gym to workout (because you are not suppose to workout when you're sick). At some point I realized that a subconscious part of me was using this as a way to get out of exercise. What I do now is I make myself still go to the gym (unless I'm throwing up).I may not have the crazy good workout that I usually have, but the act of just getting there and doing some sort of workout lets me know that the excuse is not working. I might as well not use it.

Occasionally, we don't realize we are putting things off, but we are making excuses. Weeks or months may go by before you realize you didn't take any action towards what you've wanted to do. It's a natural and normal tendency to find excuses. But you can overcome them!

Are any of your excuses good excuses? If so, how can you work around them? Most of us have excuses of some sort and sometimes they are just lame excuses and sometimes they are valid.

Be honest with yourself about which one it is. Lame excuses are just a way for you to avoid what you need to do. A justifiable excuse is something that is truly a challenge, but can still be worked around!

If your feet, ankles or knees hurt, Go workout upper body that day. Kayaking can give a great cardio workout without the strain on the lower body. If your upper body is sore then maybe a lower body weight day is in order. If you are tired then just go on a walk. At least you are keeping with the time commitment of your workouts.

There are ways around most challenges that life throws at us, it is our job to find a creative solution to what comes up.

What are some excuses you use? Are they good reasons not to do something or just a way for you to avoid doing what you need to do?

_____
_____
_____
_____
_____
_____
_____
_____
_____
_____
_____
_____
_____
_____
_____

Resist Temptation

"I generally avoid temptation unless I can't resist it"~ Mae West

This is a huge one for me. I tend to have issues resisting certain foods so I keep them out of the house. That way if I really want some chocolate I have to go out to a chocolate shop to get a piece.

Many of us have issues with food. This seems to be one of the biggest barriers to our health goals.

Sometimes it is an emotional eating issue. And being aware is half the battle.

Emotional eating is something many of us do, but contrary to popular belief we do not succumb to emotional eating only when we are sad, mad or depressed, but also when we are happy, bored, etc.

We can emotional eat for any mood. We sometimes have different foods we crave depending on the moods. I know that I can crave chocolate worse when I am super happy, because I want to celebrate.

Emotional hunger usually comes on instantly, where as

normal hunger is usually more of a gradual thing. Now I say usually because I know for me many times my normal hunger can come on instantly.

Another thing I like to do is look at what I want to eat. Generally for me if something healthy and lean is looking good then I am genuinely hungry, if I only want cookies and sweet things or cheeses then chances are I am hungry out of emotional needs.

If you are having emotional hunger, then do some other activity. Some exercise is great if you are in a position to do so. Many of our habits can be linked to emotions so understanding this and having a plan of action when they come up can help tremendously.

Have a plan for when these issues arise. First line of defense is to drink a big glass of water to make sure you are not just thirsty. If you are still having cravings have a cup of tea, some gum, some carrot sticks, have an apple or even go for a walk.

I also like to find healthy alternatives to what I like, be it healthy desserts, or dishes. Like stevia sweetened chocolate.

Make a list for yourself and have these healthy alternatives available and easy to access. Keep the bad choices out of the house or harder to access.

What Cravings really get you off track?

_____
_____
_____
_____
_____
_____
_____
_____
_____
_____

What are some good alternatives to your cravings?

_____
_____
_____
_____
_____
_____
_____
_____
_____
_____

Have Patience with Yourself

"Why is patience so important?"

"Because it makes us pay attention."

~ Paulo Coelho

I know this one all too well. I tend to want to push and push even if my body is tired. Guess what? Your body will push back.

In the past I have had health issues that have kept me from getting where I wanted to be. It can be frustrating. We must be our own best friend and be understanding. When you show patience with yourself, you are showing yourself love. You are also letting yourself know that you will get to your ultimate goal. It just may take time and some trial and error.

Since society tells us to look for quick fixes it's easy to make the mistake of giving up to soon, say after you have failed perhaps 1-5 times. That's the "normal" thing to do. But what could have happened if someone just kept going after that? And for each failure learned more and more about what works for them? Maybe the 8th or 10th time is when they would have succeeded. I would be willing to do something 10 times or even 20 or 50 times if I knew I would eventually succeed. Wouldn't you?

I think people often make a mistake of giving up too early. Your mind probably has a reasonable time frame for success. This might not correspond to a realistic time frame though. And that's not to say that you should do the same thing over and over in exactly the same manner. It's better to do it differently and keep testing it out until you get the result you want.

This is a very important thing to keep in mind when it comes to personal development (healthy lifestyle) and life. Because things may not always go as planned. You could fail. You could bail out because of fear. You could become confused. You might do things you know you shouldn't have done. You could even do these things more than once. The important thing is to not stay down. Get back up and keep going until you achieve what you set out to do!

What common things do you get impatient with yourself on? List them and then think of how you can be nicer to yourself in the future.

_____
_____
_____
_____
_____

Part 4

Things To Think About!

Theory vs. Reality

"An oak and a reed were arguing about their strength. When a strong wind came up, the reed avoided being uprooted by bending and leaning with the gusts of wind. But the oak stood firm and was torn up by the roots." ~Aesop

*I*t will always be different in theory than in actuality, so leave wiggle room.

This one is so true for most of us in life. We always think, "Well, I planned it out so this is exactly how it should go, right?" Not usually.

Sometimes it really does happen just as we planned, but in my experience that is very seldom. There are always more plans than we know in store for us. Leave a little wiggle room in your plans for the unexpected and stay open to other possibilities. You never know where they could take you!

A common one that happens often to people is with their jobs. Many people plan to stay at their secure jobs and work really hard make it to a certain level in the company and then retire at 50 or 60. But what happens to so many people is that suddenly the company has a downgrade or they decide to bring in younger cheaper labor. You suddenly get laid off. It was unexpected, you did not plan for this. But you start looking around at other jobs and find your dream job that you did not know even existed, or maybe you decide to go into business for yourself. This is a better outcome than you could have even planned for. How we think it will work out and how it does is sometimes light years apart in similarity, but you still got where you would like to be, so be easy on how you will get where you want to go.

Think of an event in your life that did not go as planned, but in the long run turned out to be a much better result!

_____
_____
_____
_____
_____
_____
_____
_____
_____
_____

Whenever you are upset because things are not going the way you planned think about this event and remember that sometimes it can wind up being better than you originally thought!

Fly Wheel Effect

"Success requires first expending ten units of effort to produce one unit of results. Your momentum will then produce ten units of results with each unit of effort"

~ Charles J. Givens

$\mathcal{A}$ fly wheel takes a lot of effort to move. You can push and push and push and it may budge so little that it is unperceivable.

When you keep pushing and keep pushing, it starts to move a bit, and then a bit more, and a bit more until eventually it has picked up momentum. It eventually reaches a point where it is moving at such a speed that it is moving under its own weight and keeping itself rolling with very little effort from you.

The fly wheel effect applies to anything we do in life.

You start on your exercise and eating right today, but you are not seeing the changes. You keep on the path and pretty soon you are seeing some small changes in your body, maybe a slight amount of increased energy.

You keep pushing this fly wheel and the changes are becoming a little more noticeable. People are complimenting you. Your increased energy is much more noticeable.

You keep on with this and after a while you have your habit engrained, you are enjoying healthy food, you have a ton of energy and you body is looking amazing.

Once you are at the point of this becoming habit, the ball is rolling under its own momentum, and all you have to do is stay on for the ride!

We commonly see this when we are starting a new career. At first it is taking a ton of effort to learn all the ins and outs of the job and we are not being very effecient. But as we stick with the job longer and longer we start to learn exactly what we need to do and then many parts of the job become unconscious. Then it is just a matter of staying on for the ride.

The same thing happens in may parts of our life. It takes a lot of effort at first, but eventually it is rolling smoothly and you can not remember why it was so hard to get started in the first place.

Silver Linings are Everywhere

"Within every setback or obstacle there lies the seed of an equal or greater opportunity or benefit"~ Napoleon Hill

Embrace problems and grow from them, finding solutions for the problems that arise can open up so many great opportunities.

How many times have you been in a situation and you thought it was just the worst thing that could have ever happened and then a week, a month or a year later you realize it was a blessing in disguise?

Find the lessons, possibilities or blessings in these life events earlier. If you can not find the positive in the situation then just know that it is happening for a reason and that the reason for it will eventually show itself.

This especially goes for health and fitness. We can sprain something; have issues with our food etc. The trick is to see what the challenge is, how you can overcome the issue, and what the gift is from that problem.

For instance, let's say you normally run for cardio and you wind up having a knee problem and have to avoid running for a month or two and you decide to swim in the mean time. You then discover that you really love swimming and have a natural knack for it. Maybe you decide to compete in swimming because of this. You would have never known that you were good at swimming if that knee problem had not come about.

What are you learning? Sometimes it is even just as simple as teaching you to be stronger and more resilient or to be more patient.

I could tell you so many stories of things that I thought were complete disasters and later on turned out to the best thing that could have happened and in some cases actually saved my life. Trust that everything happens for a reason and look for the seed of good in the "problem".

What we want to do here is see the silver lining in these events sooner. It may not even be the greater good of the event but just some good seed within this event.

I remember driving home from another city with a friend of mine and as we were getting close to home my car broke down, I looked at her and smiled, I said "this is great!"

I know she thought I was crazy. But I explained that we are so close to home, this is so much better than if we would have broken down on the highway.

` How about a common one. Road rage. What if you are on the road and some jerk cuts you off and is acting like a fool. The silver lining in this could be to remember not to act like this. Or it could be that they just reminded you how good your life really is.

What bad event have you dealt with lately, and what was the silver lining of it?

_____

_____

_____

_____

_____

_____

_____

_____

_____

_____

_____

_____

_____

_____

_____

Search for the silver linings in as many situations as possible. Trust me, they are everywhere!

You are in Charge

"The question isn't who is going to let me; it's who is going to stop me."~ Ayn Rand

One of the most powerful things to realize in our lives is that we are in charge of everything! What we eat, how much money we make, how we look. We are in charge of everything in our lives.

A great way to use this is by realizing that you are in charge, not your cravings, not your laziness. Say it out loud.

"I AM IN CHARGE!"

When you truly believe this, you will be amazed at what you can overcome and what you can resist. This is taking responsibility for your own life. When you take responsibility for your life you will realize you can do anything you want. You simply have to want it.

Focusing on solutions comes in very handy in combination with this technique. This way you can look at your health and if it is not what you think it should be, then acknowledge that you are in charge of the health you have. You can then look for the solutions to get the health you want.

But you must take action!

Finding solutions and sitting on them does you no good. You must take action and create the better health you desire and deserve. **YOU ARE IN CHARGE!**

If you feel like you have no control of your eating, that it is out of control. The first thing you have to recognize that where you are at is all up to you. No one else is forcing you to eat certain foods. The next step is using the solutions portion. You are in charge of what you keep in the house, you are in charge of the meals you prep and the meals you pack. As you do this you are taking control over the eating issues. You use the solutions to put in place some better habits around the food and before you know it you feel good about what you are creating.

If you are really out of shape and have been blaming lack of time for it, the first thing you have to do is understand you made this choice. Your fitness has not been a priority. This was no ones choice but yours. Then you can look at what you have control over. You could not spend so much time online and use that time for the gym, you can not work so much overtime, you could do a workout at lunch or even do 10 minute segments of workouts. These are your choices. And sometimes they are hard choices. Do you keep the overtime and make more money or do you take that time to get yourself in better shape? What ever you choose is fine, but you can not blame anyone else for your lack of fitness it is your choice and your choice alone.

I know that this can be a hard one for many to swallow. It is difficult to look at a life situation that we do not want and admit that it is our choice, but it is worth it. The power you gain over your life and your future vastly outweighs the pain of having to take the credit for everything.

What did you think in the past you had no control over? What solutions can you put in place to show you are in charge?

_____
_____
_____
_____
_____
_____
_____
_____
_____
_____

Starting Over

"The greatest glory in living lies not in never falling, but in rising every time we fall."
- Nelson Mandela

Start at the beginning whenever you need to.

Sometimes we get off track. Maybe we were doing really well with eating great and working out regularly and then we get overwhelmed and things start to fall apart.

Life gets busy and sometimes we need to stop what we are doing and figure out how to start back up so we can get back to where we were.

There are times in my life where things get too hectic and my workouts and eating can start to suffer. I will be eating more chocolate than usual, or eating out more than I should. That is when I stop what I am doing and look at what I need to do to get back on track. I start back at the beginning. Even if you have to start back with small, slow steps, at least you are back on the path. The most important part here is to remember this is a journey not a destination; we have set backs at times. The setbacks do not determine your success and character, how you handle them and getting back up, does.

Remember!

No matter what habit you decide you want to make a part of your life, it is of the utmost importance to have fun while you're doing it. If you're having fun, it's more likely the habit will stick because it's something you enjoy doing.

And, as always, remember to

LIVE FULL OUT!

About Author

I never thought I would be a writer. Not in a million years. I did not believe it was my talent. But I have so much information that I want to share and want to be able to help more people, so I started. I figured this is one of the best ways to help more people at once. What you read is my first book, I have 2 more already on the way. I get better at detail and explanations with each day I write.

I started on this path because of my own health and fitness issues. I began to have others ask me questions to help them with their health and it just continued from there. I have been involved in health since then. It has been 18 years now that I have been involved and 12 years since I have been certified in the health and fitness industry.

My desire to help others with their health and motivation came from dealing with a plethora of health issues and abuse. From an early age I dealt with allergies and bad body image issues which resulted in anorexia and then weight gain. I have also dealt with blood sugar issues and other issues that would get in the way of my exercise. I have been through abuse at the hands of someone who supposedly loved me. This taught me a great deal and I learned to love myself and do what is right for me. Too many of us berate ourselves for what we are not instead of looking at what we have done with our lives and what we have that is wonderful. And I guarantee you, you have something, more likely many things about you that are wonderful.

Through all of this I have learned to strive to always be in better health yet love myself the way I am now. It is not about being perfect, it is about working towards being a better you. I really do believe that our health is meant to support us in our daily adventures and when we look at it that way we will get to a realistic place with our health. The point is to find our way of better health that we can live with for life, not a yo yo diet. I also believe that life is too short and we should go after what we want in life. Staring death in the face a few times has given me the desire to really live full out. Hard times like these can either defeat us or they can grow us. We can grow to be more than we ever knew we could. I use what has happened in my life to fuel my ambition and to create a happier life. After all, life is too short not to live it.

Always *LIVE FULL OUT!*

Author Contact info

I love to hear from my community, if this book has helped you or if you have questions or comments. Feel free to email me.

Lauren Denos

Lauren@DynamicFitnessSystems.com

.J

www.ingramcontent.com/pod-product-compliance
Lightning Source LLC
Chambersburg PA
CBHW070601290526
45790CB00002B/741

9781482567779